GERD N

Tips on Hou

Acid Reflu

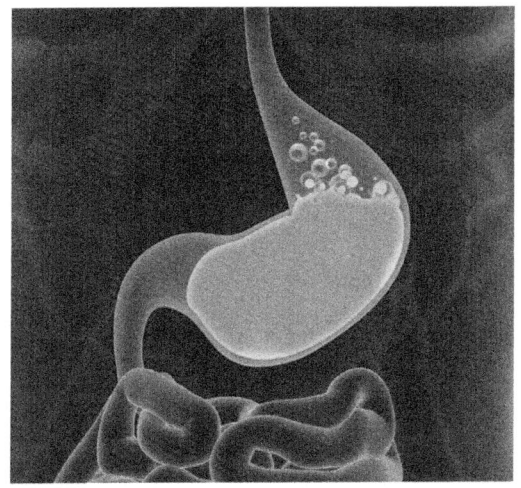

Paolo Jose de Luna

Copyright 2015 by Content Arcade Publishing

All rights reserved.

The publication is sold with the idea that the publisher is not required to render an accounting, officially permitted, or otherwise, qualified services. If advice is necessary, legal or professional, a practiced individual in the profession should be ordered.

From a Declaration of Principles which was accepted and approved equally by a Committee of the American Bar Association and a Committee of Publishers and Associations. In no way is it legal to reproduce, duplicate, or transmit any part of this document in either electronic means or printed format. Recording of this publication is strictly prohibited, and any storage of this document is not allowed unless with written permission from the publisher.

The information provided herein is stated to be truthful and consistent, in that any liability, in terms of inattention or otherwise, by any usage or abuse of any policies, processes, or directions contained within is the solitary and utter responsibility of the recipient reader. Under no circumstances will any legal responsibility or blame be held against the publisher for any reparation, damages, or monetary loss due to the information herein, either directly or indirectly.

The information herein is offered for informational purposes solely and is universal as so. The presentation of the information is without a contract or any type of guarantee. The trademarks that are used are without any consent, and the publication of the trademark is without permission or backing by the trademark owner. All trademarks and brands within this book are for clarifying purposes only and are owned by the owners themselves, not affiliated with this document.

Table of Contents

Introduction i
CHAPTER 1: 1
Understanding GERD 1
    Risk Factors 6
    Factors that May Increase the Chance of Developing GERD 8

CHAPTER 2: 12
How to Identify GERD 12
    Signs and Symptoms of GERD 12

CHAPTER 3: 17
GERD Complications 17

CHAPTER 4: 23
How to Diagnose GERD 23
    Laboratory Examinations 23

CHAPTER 5: 27
How to Manage and Treat GERD 27
    GERD Management and Treatment 27
        Dietary and Lifestyle Changes 29
    Over-the-Counter and Prescription Medications 33
        Natural Remedies 36
Conclusion 41

Introduction

Today, many people experience what is commonly known as heartburn. Other terms that are usually interchanged with heartburn include acid indigestion, pyrosis, and acid reflux. The main symptom of pyrosis is a burning pain and discomfort in the patient's chest, stomach, and sometimes in the throat and mouth. It feels like there is a burning fire in the patient's chest. This is usually as a result of gastric or acid reflux, a condition that occurs when stomach acid flows back into the food pipe. The acidic contents of the stomach cause a burning pain and irritation as they pass through the esophagus.

Acid reflux is one of the key symptoms of **Gastroesophageal Reflux Disease**, which is commonly known as GERD. It can also happen to those suffering from heart disease. GERD is a digestive disorder that causes a lot of pain in the chest and makes the patient feel uncomfortable. People who suffer from the condition usually complain of a burning sensation in their chest and end up looking for medical attention including admission to hospital for treatment.

However, some of the people who suffer from GERD choose to seek medication and stay at home. The bottom line is that many GERD patients try to manage the condition at home. Others may have to stay at the hospital if necessary. Not every GERD patient ends up spending several days in the hospital after consulting a physician. If a GERD patient complains of severe pain and the doctor determines that the patient has gastric ulcers or an infection, the doctor may recommend hospitalization. The doctor may also find it necessary to admit a patient with the symptoms of heartburn and heart disease.

It is important to do a proper diagnosis to determine the real cause of the problem and determine whether the patient's complaint is related to GERD or a heart problem. This is important for the doctor to make the necessary arrangements for treatment.

GERD is a common health problem affecting the gastrointestinal (GI) tract. Just like other health conditions affecting the GI tract, it is not difficult to find the appropriate treatment option for the patient. Also, people suffering from GERD can choose from a wide selection of methods to treat or manage the condition. One popular intervention for GERD patients involves the use of different dietary plans. Persons suffering from GERD can also prevent and manage GERD by modifying their lifestyle habits.

Like any other health problem, GERD is associated with various risk factors. A risk factor refers to something that can increase the chances of developing a disease. In the field of health and medicine, the first important step in the disease prevention process is to understand the potential risk factors. With adequate information about the risk factors associated with GERD, it is easy to prevent the disorder and reduce the chances of medication or hospitalization. Several factors may contribute to the development of GERD, but the most common causes include regular consumption of highly acidic substances or foods including coffee, carbonated beverages, and alcohol.

If these risk factors are not addressed and the doctor's diagnosis proves that the patient has GERD, the next step is to use the appropriate treatment and management methods. Without proper treatment or management in the early stages of development, GERD can cause various complications. Persons suffering from this digestive disorder are also at a greater risk of developing other health problems including duodenal ulcers, gastritis, and gastric ulcers.

It is important for those suffering from GERD to seek medical attention. However, it helps to understand the key indicators of the problem as well as the recommended treatment and management methods to help the patient at home. Abdominal pain is often a major symptom of GERD and can be managed at home the patient knows the appropriate steps. In addition to experiencing acid reflux, patients with GERD may vomit or feel nauseated.

The right treatment and management methods seek to reduce or eliminate these symptoms. When it comes to prevention, it is easy to prevent the disorder by making the lifestyle changes discussed in this book. If you decide to modify your lifestyle habits, you will prevent GERD and reduce the risk of developing other health conditions. Generally, people with GERD can benefit from various management methods and the good news is that GED is easy to manage.

This book focuses on everything you need to know about GERD. This includes a definition of the disorder, its signs, and the symptoms exhibited by GERD patients. Prevention is always better than cure and that's why we will talk about the different ways of preventing GERD. Apart from that, we will also discuss the recommended management methods to help GERD patients better manage the condition. Some of these methods can be used at home without having to visit the hospital all the time.

By the end of the book, you will learn how to manage the GERD using simple methods while at home. Let's get started!

CHAPTER 1:

Understanding GERD

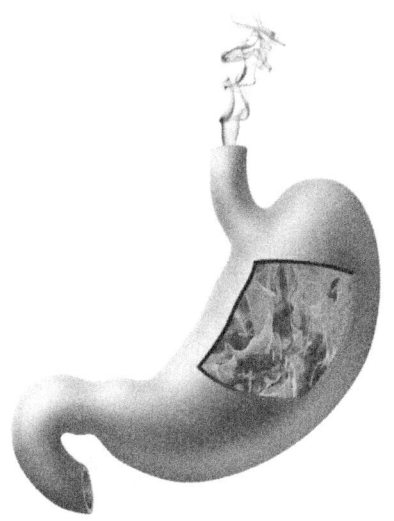

Gastroesophageal Reflux Disease (GERD) is a digestive disorder that occurs when the acidic contents of the stomach or duodenum flow back into the esophagus. The content flows backward and goes through the food pipe. There is a substantial amount of acid contained in the stomach or duodenal content, which causes patients to develop various signs and symptoms. As the acid starts to flow through the food pipe, it causes a burning sensation in the patient's chest and esophagus. The burning pain can also be felt along the patient's neck. This makes the patient feel uncomfortable and often prompts medical attention to relieve the irritation.

A patient with GERD may have several signs and symptoms including heartburn, nausea, epigastric pain, vomiting, regurgitation, and dizziness. These are the key symptoms doctors look for to properly diagnose the disorder. Although GERD is a digestive disorder that affects the GI tract, it is a normal occurrence among young people and adults as longs as it does not happen frequently. The disorder develops due to various causes and risk factors.

Fortunately, it's possible to prevent GERD from developing by addressing some of the common risk factors. Most of the known risk factors are associated with an individual's lifestyle habits. You can change bad lifestyle habits to healthy habits if you are determined to prevent GERD from occurring. If you take the necessary prevention steps, then you don't have to waste time on treatment and management.

As mentioned earlier, GERD is characterized by a burning pain that makes the affected person feel uncomfortable. However, the nature of the discomfort may vary from one person to another depending on several factors. For instance, it can be extremely uncomfortable for people who are experiencing it firsthand. Luckily, it is easy to control the disorder and even treat it at home. The most important thing is to know the signs, do a proper diagnosis, and know what to do if the patient is comfortable at home.

If you decide to treat or manage GERD at home, it is important to choose the right interventions. Careless interventions won't help and some of them might worsen the situation and probably cause serious complications. So, if you are determined to treat the condition at home, it is advisable to have the right information.

You need to get in touch with a doctor to make sure you are treating GERD. This is a vital step because the symptoms of GERD could also signify a different health problem. For instance, people who complain of heartburn, which is one of the key symptoms of GERD, may be suffering from other health problems such as myocardial infarction and heart failure. Of course, you don't want to end up using the wrong treatment methods or keeping a heart disease patient at home without knowing the looming danger.

It is difficult to succeed in treating a patient without a clear idea of what they are suffering from. The best way to make sure the patient receives the right treatment is to do an accurate assessment of their signs and symptoms. A diagnosis is needed to accurately assess the problem. Once a proper diagnosis is done and it's evident that the patient has GERD, it is easy to rule out other conditions before concluding that the disorder can be treated at home.

There are several health conditions with the same signs and symptoms as GERD. This means that, in addition to having GERD, the patient could be having other correlated health problems that need the attention of a professional health practitioner. After the diagnosis, the doctor may find it necessary to admit the patient. If the patient is complaining of chest pain in the epigastric area, they could be suffering from myocardial infarction or heart attack. These health conditions need to be ruled out and that is why it's advisable to perform clinical examinations.

Many hospitals carry out the necessary procedures to confirm whether or not the patient is suffering from heart disease or any other health problem with the same signs and symptoms as GERD. The most important thing is to contact a doctor and do a diagnosis if you intend to treat GERD at home to avoid unnecessary complications.

So, what makes the stomach's acidic contents flow into the esophagus? The first possible cause of the problem is a weak esophageal sphincter. Secondly, the problem may occur if the esophageal sphincter relaxes inappropriately. Food enters the stomach through the lower esophageal sphincter (LES). The LES is made up of muscles that open to allow the food to enter the stomach. Once the food or fluid enters the stomach, the LES closes to prevent gastric acid and other stomach contents from moving backward. The backward movement of stomach contents with gastric acid causes heartburn in the esophagus.

GERD develops when the LES fails to perform its function properly. In patients with GERD, the LES weakens and its muscles are no longer able to hold tightly to prevent the stomach's acidic contents from flowing backward into the esophagus. The stomach's contents may eventually reach the throat and oral cavity. When this happens, the patient is likely to vomit. Persons with this problem may also display other symptoms including a burning sensation in the chest and throat.

The burning sensation experienced by people with GERD is what is commonly known as heartburn. Just like the acidic solutions we know, the acid can burn the human body. This explains why there is a burning feeling as the stomach's acidic contents pass through the esophagus and throat. Those suffering from GERD often complain of heartburn and regurgitation.

Now let's talk about the figures to understand the prevalence of GERD. According to the available data, there are 15 million GERD patients in every 60 million individuals. This data refers to the number of people who experience heartburn or GERD every day. However, some people are more likely to develop GERD depending on their current condition or age. Research has shown that the most susceptible people are children and expectant women. However, it is easy to manage the condition at home, so they don't need to be hospitalized.

According to some studies, all children including infants are at a higher risk of developing GERD compared to the rest of the population. Children who develop the disorder may show various symptoms including vomiting and coughing. Others may develop respiratory problems. If you notice serious symptoms, consult your doctor immediately for more advice.

Risk Factors

A risk factor is something that increases the chances of developing a health condition. When it comes to GERD, some people are more susceptible to the disorder compared to other people due to certain risk factors. The most common risk factors often weaken the lower esophageal sphincter allowing gastric acid to flow from the stomach into your esophagus. In addition to weakening the LES, some risk factors can increase the level of acid in the stomach. When the amount of acid reaches abnormally high levels and the gastric content start to flow backward through the esophagus, the patient begins to experience a burning sensation and feels uncomfortable. Several factors can contribute to the development of GERD. The most common risk factors include:

- **Being obese or overweight** – Obesity is a complex disorder characterized by excessive amounts of body fat. People who are obese or overweight are at a higher risk of developing a wide range of health problems including high blood pressure and diabetes mellitus. These people also have higher chances of developing GERD than people with normal body weight. They are prone to GERD because their stomach and esophageal lining are under pressure. This increases the chances of having acid reflux.

- **Pregnancy** – Expectant women are usually susceptible to a variety of health problems and GERD is one of those problems. The developing fetus in the womb exerts pressure on the abdomen. The pressure can push the stomach's acidic content into the esophagus. The chances of developing GERD during pregnancy are high during the last 2 trimesters.

- **Hiatal Hernia** – Hiatal hernia is a condition that occurs when the upper part of the stomach pushes into the chest cavity through a small opening (hiatus) in the diaphragm. As the upper section of the stomach pushes through the diaphragm, it exerts pressure on the stomach. As a result, the stomach's acidic content might flow back into the esophagus increasing the risk of developing GERD.

- **Slow stomach emptying** – Sometimes it takes a long time for food to empty from the stomach. When this happens, the affected person has a greater risk of developing GERD because the acidic content of the stomach can easily flow backward through the esophagus. The acid leads to the burning sensation and discomfort associated with GERD.

- **Scleroderma and other connective tissue disorders** – In human anatomy, connective tissue refers to the fibrous, elastic, fatty or cartilaginous tissue that connects and supports other tissues and organs. This type of tissue is an important building block of the esophagus and can be affected by connective tissue problems like scleroderma. Those suffering from scleroderma have tight and hard connective tissues or skin. If the esophagus is affected by such a condition, it may not close properly when drinking or eating. This means that the acidic content of the stomach can easily flow backward through the esophagus.

Factors that May Increase the Chance of Developing GERD

In addition to the abovementioned risk factors, other factors may also increase the chances of developing GERD or heartburn. These factors may either cause the muscles of the esophagus to relax or increase the level of acid in the stomach. Other factors may cause indigestion, which is also known as dyspepsia. Indigestion can cause gastric contents to flow back into the esophagus leading to a burning pain and discomfort in the chest area. Other factors that can lead to GERD are as follows:

- **Smoking** — Studies have linked cigarette smoking to GERD with findings showing that smokers suffer from constant acid reflux. According to doctors, nicotine tends to relax the smooth muscles of the lower esophageal sphincter. As the muscles relax, the acidic content of the stomach may flow back into the esophagus. Smoking also leads to GERD by reducing salivation, increasing acid secretion in the stomach, interfering with the functions of the esophageal muscles, and damaging the esophageal lining. Saliva contains bicarbonate, a substance that can neutralize stomach acid to reduce the effects of acid reflux or GERD. Smokers have less ability to neutralize the acid because they generally produce less saliva than nonsmokers.

- **Dry mouth** — Dry mouth is a problem that occurs when the salivary glands are unable to produce enough saliva. If your mouth is dry, you don't have sufficient amounts of bicarbonate in your saliva to neutralize the stomach's acidic content.

- **Food with excessive fats** – High-fat foods are considered to be trigger foods because they can lead to the development of GERD. These foods can trigger heartburn by relaxing the lower esophageal sphincter. Foods with high amounts of fat can also stimulate the release of cholecystokinin (CCK), a peptide hormone that may relax the lower esophageal sphincter leading to acid reflux. CCK may also lead to delayed stomach emptying, which is another risk factor for GERD.

- **Caffeine** – Research findings have revealed that caffeine can be a risk factor for GERD whether it's consumed in coffee or caffeinated products. Although research in this area is inconclusive, some studies have shown that the amount of caffeine found in coffee can relax the lower esophageal sphincter increasing the chances of experiencing heartburn and acid reflux.

- **Carbonated beverages and sodas** – Evidence from one study shows a significant link between carbonated soft drinks and nighttime heartburn. In another study, the risk of developing acid reflux and heartburn symptoms is higher in people who take carbonated drinks.

- **Alcohol** – Alcohol can also cause the symptoms of heartburn especially when taken in large amounts. It can contribute to heartburn by relaxing the lower esophageal sphincter or by increasing the level of acid in the stomach. Excessive alcohol can also damage the esophageal lining making the esophagus more sensitive to gastric acid.

- **Asthma** – People with asthma have higher chances of developing GERD than those without the disease. Research has shown that most adults suffering from asthma also have GERD. Asthma may trigger GERD and the vice versa is also true. Asthma causes pressure changes in the chest and abdomen. When the lungs swell, the stomach is exposed to a lot of pressure and this might cause the muscles responsible for preventing acid reflux to relax. Consequently, stomach acid flows up into the esophagus.

- **Diabetes mellitus** – Some researchers have found out that people with diabetes mellitus are at a higher risk of developing GERD than people without the condition. Those suffering from diabetes mellitus suffer various complications including esophageal dysfunction. The most common problems among these patients include weak esophageal contractions, reduced peristalsis velocity, fewer peristaltic waves, abnormal gastroesophageal reflux, and low pressure in the lower esophageal sphincter. Abnormal gastroesophageal reflux simply refers to GERD.

As you can see, there is a significant number of risk factors that are directly linked to one's lifestyle habits. For this reason, one of the best ways to prevent GERD is to make lifestyle changes. It's also evident that some foods may increase the likelihood to develop GERD, so the disorder can be prevented by making dietary changes. If the development of GERD is not prevented, then the patient can choose from several treatment options. The main goal of treating the disorder is to neutralize the stomach's acidic content, protect the esophagus from stomach acids, and prevent the triggers of acid reflux and heartburn.

If you are suffering from chronic GERD, it's advisable to consult with your physician. This is vital because you could be suffering from other health conditions. Your doctor needs to rule out other health problems with the same symptoms as GERD by performing the appropriate tests. It is important to make sure you are not suffering from other health conditions before you begin the treatment process.

CHAPTER 2:

How to Identify GERD

Gastroesophageal reflux disease

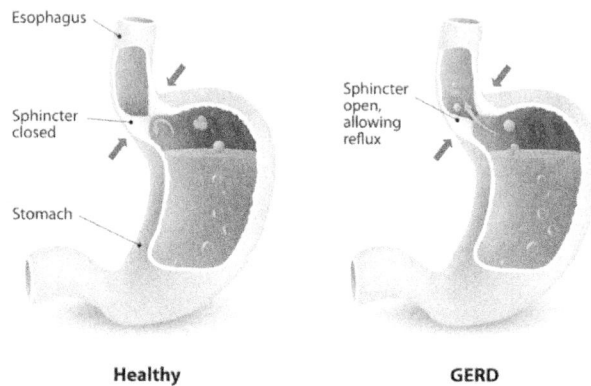

Healthy **GERD**

Signs and Symptoms of GERD

The first step of an effective treatment process is to identify the known signs and symptoms of the disorder. However, the assessment should be done with caution because GERD has the same symptoms as other health disorders. For example, a person with GERD may have the same symptoms as someone with heart disease. We've already mentioned that other conditions must be ruled out to make sure the patient is suffering from GERD. There are several steps including taking into account the patient's health history. In some cases, the patient may have other health problems with similar or the same symptoms as GERD. The most important thing is to ensure that the assessment is accurate before the patient starts the treatment and management process.

We've already talked about heartburn and it's important to explain it in detail because most of the people who suffer from GERD usually complain of heartburn. Simply put, heartburn or pyrosis is the burning pain or sensation experienced when the acidic contents of the stomach flow back into the esophagus. When the gastric content of the stomach starts to flow through the esophagus, you will experience a heat. Patients with this digestive system disorder are also likely to develop other health problems. If the condition remains untreated for a long time, the patient might develop esophagitis.

To properly identify GERD and any other health disorder, it is important to know the signs and symptoms. Here is a list of the signs and symptoms of GERD:

- **Heartburn or pyrosis** – This is the burning pain or discomfort experienced in the chest area or throat when the acidic contents of the stomach are forced back up into the esophagus.
- **Indigestion or dyspepsia** – Persons with dyspepsia experience pain or discomfort in the upper abdominal area. They also experience a burning sensation, nausea, burping, and bloating.
- **Regurgitation** – Regurgitation is the expulsion of undigested food from the esophagus.

- **Dysphagia and odynophagia** – People with dysphagia have difficulty swallowing certain foods as well as liquids. In extreme cases, they may not be able to swallow anything at all because of pain in the throat or esophagus. Odynophagia is characterized by pain in the mouth, throat or esophagus upon swallowing.
- **Excessive salivation** – If the salivary glands are producing excessive amounts of saliva, it could be a sign of GERD.
- **Esophagitis** – Patients with esophagitis have an inflamed esophagus which is caused by the acidic contents of the stomach. The inflammation damages the esophagus leading to chest pain and swallowing problems.
- **Nausea and vomiting** – Nausea is a stomach discomfort that makes you want to vomit. It usually happens before vomiting.
- **Chest pain** – In addition to the burning sensation experienced in the chest, a person with GERD may experience pain in the sternum.
- **Abdominal pain** – Pain in the abdomen is also a possible sign of GERD. Those suffering from the disorder may experience pain in the epigastric area of their stomach. Abdominal pain may eventually radiate to the patient's chest area and esophageal lining.
- Appetite loss
- Fatigue
- Dizziness
- Lightheadedness

Pain in the chest area is one of the alarming signs of GERD and most people tend to misinterpret it as a sign of a heart attack. This happens even among people who have never suffered from cardiac disease. As indicated earlier in this book, the best thing to do is to perform an accurate assessment to rule out the possibility of having other diseases other than GERD before treatment begins.

It is important to keep in mind that those suffering from GERD may not have the same symptoms. The symptoms can vary from one person to another depending on several factors. Some patients will only complain of a burning pain in their chest or along their esophagus. There are also GERD patients who don't display any symptoms of pyrosis. Patients who don't experience a burning feeling in their chest or esophagus may display the other signs of GERD including appetite loss, vomiting, nausea, dyspepsia or indigestion, and lightheadedness.

When looking for the signs and symptoms of any health problem, we usually want to know how frequent and how severe the problem is. When it comes to GERD, experts say that the best way to determine whether a heartburn is severe or not is to look at its frequency or the number of occurrences within a certain duration. If there is enough evidence of frequent acid reflux, the affected individual should consult a doctor as soon as possible. The doctor will perform the necessary clinical tests to find out whether the acid reflux is a sign of GERD or another health problem. With a proper assessment of the condition, the patient can start treatment as early as possible depending on what the doctor thinks needs to be done after the assessment.

GERD MANAGEMENT

If the test results indicate that the heartburn is a sign of GERD, the doctor may recommend a variety of treatment methods to relieve the symptoms. If you have GERD, there is no need to worry because this digestive disorder can be resolved within a very short time. Another good thing about the disorder is that it is easy to manage with remedies that are easy to find. For instance, you can easily manage GERD at home if you know the recommended natural remedies or medications that can be purchased from the local drugstore. Depending on the severity of the condition, you don't have to stay at the hospital. However, it is always important to look for a doctor's advice before using any form of treatment for GERD. It is for your own safety because you don't want to end up using remedies or treatments that will worsen your situation. Another benefit of consulting with a doctor is that you can be sure that the treatment methods or drugs you are using are effective.

CHAPTER 3:

GERD Complications

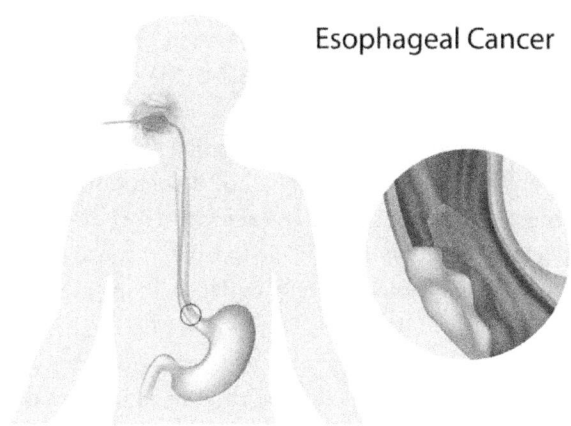

Esophageal Cancer

The good thing about health problems that affect the GI tract is that they are easy to treat. As we already know from the previous chapters of this book, it is important to consult with a physician, but you can treat and manage GI tract problems at home. If you have some useful medical knowledge to help you treat or manage your health problem, then there is no need for hospitalization. However, you should remember that sometimes the condition might worsen and go beyond what you can manage with the amount of knowledge you have. When this happens, even simple tasks can cause complications. Just like other health conditions, certain complications may arise in patients with GERD. These complications usually occur if the disorder is left untreated for a long time.

Once it is evident that the patient has GERD, it is important to start the treatment and management process immediately. Failure to treat or manage the problem can contribute to various complications. For instance, there is a possibility of having an inflamed esophagus if GERD is left untreated for a long time. Chronic cases of inflammation can cause a wide range of complications that require the attention of a professional medical practitioner. In some cases, the patient may still experience GERD despite using the remedies and treatment methods recommended by a doctor. If you realize that the treatment methods and remedies recommended by the doctor are not working, it is advisable to consult with the doctor for further advice on how to deal with the problem.

If GERD remains untreated for prolonged periods, the patient may develop several complications that need the attention of a physician. It's important to know the possible complications in order to take the necessary action if they occur. Here are some of the common complications of GERD:

- **Esophageal Strictures** – Untreated cases of GERD can lead to strictures which are characterized by scarred or damaged lining of the esophagus. In prolonged cases, cells on the walls of the lower esophageal sphincter are exposed to the stomach's acidic content causing damage to the lining. When this happens, scar tissue forms on the walls of the esophagus leading to a narrow pathway. The patient develops dysphagia meaning that it is difficult for them to swallow food or fluids. In severe cases, the patient may even experience pain when swallowing. This is what is commonly known as odynophagia. The best action to take is to seek medical attention if you notice these symptoms to avoid further complications.

- **Esophageal Ulcers** – We already know that gastric content is acidic and is the one responsible for the burning sensation experienced by persons with GERD. When the lining of the esophagus is exposed to the stomach's acidic content for a long time, the patient is likely to have a damaged esophageal lining. This happens because the tissues that make up the esophageal lining can be eroded by the acidic content of the stomach. Once the acid erodes the tissues, the patient can develop sores or ulcers. The ulcers or sores can cause several health problems including pain and bleeding. Additionally, the patient may have trouble swallowing food and fluids. If you are suffering from GERD and you have chronic pain in your chest and you find it difficult to swallow food, visit your physician immediately for advice. You should also consult your physician if you vomit and notice some bloodstains in your vomitus.

- **Barrett's Esophagus** – In cases where a GERD patient stays for a long time without seeking treatment, the esophagus may undergo significant changes due to the damage caused by the acidic content of the stomach. The changes that occur in patients with long-term or chronic GERD increase the risk of developing cancer of the esophagus. Due to prolonged exposure to acid reflux, abnormal changes take place in the lining or walls of the esophagus. Over time, the normal cells that make up the esophageal lining are replaced with other cells that are not usually found in this area. The abnormal cells that start to grow in the esophagus resemble the cells found in the small intestine. When the abnormal cells start to grow, the patient is at a higher risk of developing esophageal cancer than a GERD patient with normal esophageal cells. It might take some time to notice these changes, but it's possible. If you have GERD and the doctor suspects you have Barrett's Esophagus, the best and most common way of diagnosing the problem is to perform an endoscopy.

- **Esophageal Tumors** – Another complication that might occur in GERD patients is the development of tumors. Those suffering from chronic GERD may develop tumors along the lining of the esophageal. The smooth tissues found in this area are prone to tumors if the acidic content of the stomach causes extensive damage. Persons with esophageal tumors may have a number of complaints. Some patients have difficulty swallowing while others develop a lump or mass that can be seen on their neck, especially on their esophageal lining. Usually, the tumor is identified by performing a biopsy. An examination of the tissue helps the doctor determine whether the tumor is benign (harmless) or malignant (dangerous). Once the nature of the tumor is determined, the doctor may decide to remove the tumor through surgical procedures. The procedure can be helpful if the patient is unable to eat, drink or breathe properly.

- **Esophageal Cancer** – Cancer of the esophagus is a serious complication that can occur in GERD patients. The chances of developing this type of cancer are high if the patient has long-term GERD and does not use any form of treatment or remedy. One of the main reasons why persons with GERD are more likely to develop esophageal cancer than persons with other diseases is the chronic irritation that damages the lining of the esophagus. This explains why Barrett's Esophagus is a major risk factor for esophageal cancer. Despite its poor prognosis, esophageal cancer can be identified by conducting diagnostic examinations. The most common method of identifying the condition is to perform an endoscopic exam. During the examination, the doctor can see images of the esophageal lining and can use them to determine whether the patient is suffering from esophageal cancer.

Two types of cancers affect the esophagus: **squamous cell carcinoma** and **adenocarcinoma**. Squamous cell carcinoma begins in special cells known as squamous cells. These cells are found in the lining of the esophagus. The type of cancer that begins in these cells usually affects the middle and upper part of the esophagus. Its risk factors include alcohol abuse and smoking. Adenocarcinoma usually affects the lower area of the esophagus. It is likely to occur in patients with Barret's esophagus. The problem with esophageal cancer is that it's difficult to detect in its early stages. Those suffering from this type of cancer usually have difficulty swallowing. The esophagus continues to narrow making swallowing more difficult and sometimes painful.

So far, we already know that it is easy to manage GERD at home. However, patients with this digestive disorder should always consult a doctor before initiating any form of treatment. It is also important to seek a doctor's advice if you notice some unusual symptoms. Prolonged GERD is usually the biggest problem for those suffering from the disorder. Of course, no patient wants to end up dealing with the abovementioned complications, so it is vital to consult a professional medical practitioner. The doctor may recommend certain medications or advice the patient to make some lifestyle or dietary changes. Whatever the doctor thinks will work for you, make sure you follow the recommended steps. The best part is that you don't need a long treatment process to treat GERD. Moreover, the doctor is most likely to recommend dietary changes. This is a widely used and safe intervention for GERD patients, so you don't have to take drugs with side effects.

Since long-term GERD can lead to serious complications, you should take the appropriate steps to avoid them. You need to watch out for the signs and symptoms to identify changes that might have taken place over time. If you have been using various treatment methods for some time and the symptoms are still persistent, seek medical attention immediately. You should also consult your doctor if you notice other unusual symptoms even after taking the necessary treatments. You need to be alert when it comes to identifying the signs and symptoms because you need to identify them as early as possible. This will allow your doctor to carry out the necessary diagnostic assessments in time. You will then receive the appropriate treatment in time to reduce the risk of developing complications. You don't want to be hospitalized for something you can prevent.

CHAPTER 4:

How to Diagnose GERD

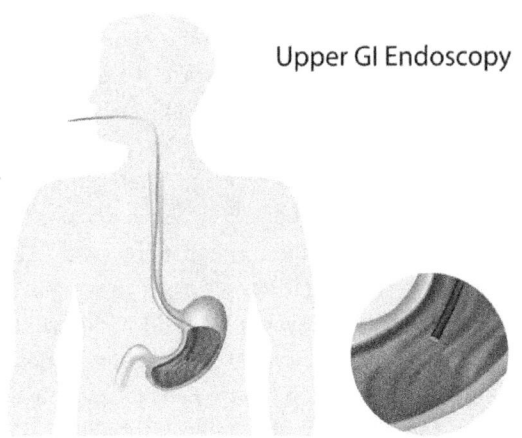

Upper GI Endoscopy

Laboratory Examinations

Just like any other health condition, the best way to know whether you are suffering from GERD is to carry out a diagnosis. If you see the signs and symptoms of GERD, you need to visit a healthcare facility for your doctor to perform the necessary tests. The doctor may use a variety of laboratory examinations and diagnostic tools to do a proper diagnosis by looking at the key indications of GERD. GERD is a gastrointestinal disorder with the same symptoms as other health problems like myocardial infarction, heart attack, gastric ulcers, gastritis, and gallbladder stones. For this reason, other health problems must be ruled out and the best way to do it is to perform a diagnosis. In most cases, doctors use the following examinations to establish whether a patient has GERD or not.

- **Upper Gastrointestinal Endoscopy** – This procedure allows the doctor to examine the lining of the esophagus and stomach. It involves inserting a thin, flexible tube with a camera and light down the throat. The light and the camera make it possible for the doctor to see and examine the lining of the esophagus for signs of GERD. An endoscopy can detect inflammation of the esophageal lining (esophagitis) and other complications. It is also a popular tool for diagnosing gastric ulcers in patients with GERD. If necessary, the doctor can collect a sample of the tissue for further examination. In a clinical setting, this procedure is known as a biopsy. The tissue sample is tested to identify Barret's esophagus and other complications associated with GERD.

- **Esophageal pH Test** – If the patient has been undergoing treatment for some time and there's no improvement, the doctor may find it necessary to carry out a pH test. Just like any other pH test, an esophageal pH test is used to measure the amount of acid in the patient's stomach. Based on the readings, the doctor can establish whether the patient has acid reflux. In some cases, the doctor may place a monitor in the patient's esophagus. The monitor could be a thin, flexible tube connected to a small computer worn around the patient's waist.

- **Esophageal Manometry** – Doctors use this test to find out if the esophagus is functioning properly. Most of the patients who suffer from GERD have trouble swallowing food and fluids. One way to establish if GERD exists is to examine the esophagus when the patient is swallowing. During the test, doctors can measure rhythmic muscle contractions in the esophagus when the patient is swallowing. The test is also used to measure the amount of pressure exerted by the esophageal lining muscles. Doctors can also use esophageal manometry to identify some GERD complications including esophageal strictures. These symptoms will help the doctor rule out other health conditions with the same signs and symptoms as GERD.

- **Upper Digestive System X-Ray** – If necessary, the doctor can take an x-ray of the patient's upper digestive system. During the procedure, the patient swallows a chalky liquid that coats the lining of the GI tract. This allows the doctor to see a silhouette of the patient's esophagus, stomach, and intestine. The doctor may also ask you to swallow a barium tablet to determine if your esophagus has narrowed.

- **Ultrasound examinations** – Ultrasound examinations make it possible to see abnormalities in the patient's esophagus, stomach, and gastrointestinal tract.

Doctors can also diagnose GERD by using other diagnostic tests including urine and blood tests. Overall, it is important to carry out laboratory examinations using the appropriate tools to make sure the patient is suffering from GERD. Also, other health conditions with similar signs and symptoms must be ruled out. Proper diagnosis means that the patient will receive the appropriate treatment.

CHAPTER 5:

How to Manage and Treat GERD

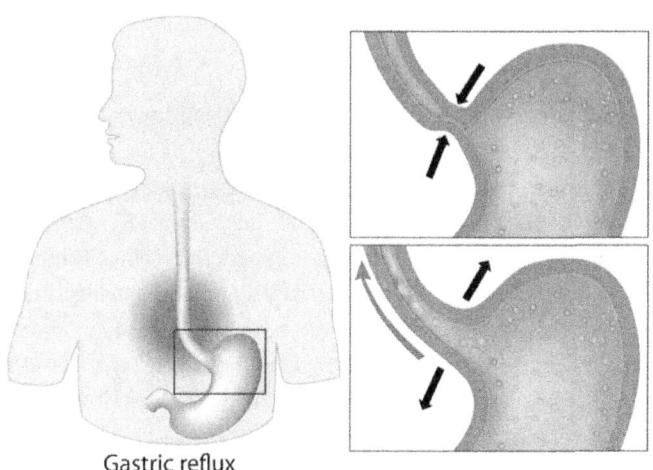

Gastric reflux

GERD Management and Treatment

So far, you've learned the various risk factors for GERD, the signs and symptoms of the disorder, the possible complications, and tests that can be done to carry out a proper diagnosis. If it's evident that the patient is suffering from GERD, the next step is to use the appropriate methods to manage or treat the problem. Luckily, it is easy to manage GERD just like other health problems that affect the GI tract. One way to manage GERD is to neutralize the acid that triggers a burning pain in the chest when gastric fluids start to flow back into the esophagus. You can neutralize it by taking some antacids, but you may not get the desired results all the time. The good news is that there are many treatment options and you can even manage GERD at home. Generally, the most important thing is to know what works best for you with the help of your doctor. You also need to do things the right way if you want to achieve the best results at the end of the treatment process.

Patients who experience regular GERD episodes often feel uncomfortable because of the symptoms. For instance, those with severe GERD may experience nausea or painful heartburn every day. Other symptoms that may occur frequently in patients with GERD include vomiting and coughing. The truth is that GERD comes with challenges that can make life almost unbearable for those suffering from the disorder. Once a proper diagnosis is done, it is important to manage the problem as soon as possible to reduce the pain. Immediate management of the disorder is also necessary to reduce the chances of developing esophageal strictures, esophageal cancer and other complications that can make life more difficult for GERD patients.

The process of treating GERD aims at achieving two key goals. The first one is to get rid of the burning pain and discomfort experienced by the patients due to frequent episodes of acid reflux and esophageal lining damage. Relieving the pain will help the patient feel more comfortable. The second goal of treating GERD is to lower the risk of developing the complications mentioned earlier in this book. As you know,

GERD patients can develop certain complications if the disorder remains untreated for a long time. Those with GERD should use the appropriate management methods to achieve both goals. With the right methods, it is easy to relieve the symptoms and improve the patient's health and overall wellbeing.

Whether you are trying to help someone else or yourself, there is a variety of methods that you can use to manage the disorder. These include lifestyle changes, dietary changes, and different types of medications. Let's look at the most common ways of managing GERD.

Dietary and Lifestyle Changes

- As mentioned earlier, being obese or overweight is a risk factor for GERD. For this reason, you should keep off fatty foods or limit foods with high amounts of fat. To reduce the risk of developing GERD or complications in people who are already suffering from the disorder, it's important to avoid extra body weight.

- Those suffering from GERD should also reduce caffeine intake. Research has shown that the amount of caffeine found in coffee, chocolate, and sodas can increase stomach acid levels. High levels of acid can damage the lining of the esophagus leading to discomfort in the affected area.
- GERD patients are also advised to limit their sugar consumption. Sweets and other sugary products can lead to high levels of gastric acid. You can reduce the

chances of experiencing acid reflux by consuming foods or products with smaller amounts of sugar.

- You already know that certain foods and drinks can increase the amount of acid in the stomach. With that in mind, GERD patients should limit citrus beverages and fruits. Just like coffee, sodas, and chocolates, citrus fruits contribute to higher levels of acid in the stomach. We know that stomach acid is responsible for damaging the lining of the esophagus in persons with GERD. If you are suffering from GERD, you want to prevent this damage and that's why it's advisable to avoid foods and drinks with citrus fruits.

- Colas, sodas, and other carbonated drinks also belong to the category of drinks that should be avoided by GERD patients. Just like citrus fruits and drinks that contain caffeine, carbonated drinks can lead to high levels of acid in the stomach. Increased levels of stomach acid can damage tissues on the walls of the esophagus leading to more complications.

- GERD patients should also avoid tomatoes and products that contain tomatoes. Just like carbonated drinks, these products can contribute to elevated levels of acid in the stomach. If you have GERD, you don't want to have more acid in your gastric fluids because the consequences can be devastating. More acid will cause more pain and damage.

- Patients with GERD should also limit pepper consumption because pepper can worsen the condition by promoting the damage caused by the stomach's acidic content. It's a well-known fact that pepper can increase pain when applied to damaged body tissues.

- Another recommended GERD management method is to stop smoking. Smokers are at a higher risk of having a weak esophageal sphincter than people who don't smoke. The esophageal sphincter opens to allow foods and fluids to enter the stomach. Once the food enters the stomach, the esophageal sphincters should close properly to prevent regurgitation. Cigarette smoking can hinder this ability, so you should avoid smoking.

- Alcohol consumption is another risk factor for GERD. If you are an alcohol user, you should limit the amount of alcohol you consume to lower the risk of having high amounts of acid in your stomach. Alcohol not only increases acid levels in the stomach but also weakens the esophageal sphincter allowing the acidic content of the stomach to flow back into the esophagus. You can avoid these problems by limiting alcohol consumption.

- Vomiting and nausea are some of the common signs and symptoms exhibited by those suffering from GERD. One way to relieve these symptoms is to eat dry crackers. The main goal of eating crackers is to prevent acidic reflux.

- One of the key goals of managing GERD is to relieve the burning sensation experienced when the stomach's acidic content flows back into the esophagus. You can achieve this goal by drinking several glasses of water.

- Another important factor to consider when managing GERD is when to eat food or drink fluids. If you have GERD, you are likely to get regurgitated during sleep. For that reason, you should eat or drink as early as possible, preferably more than two hours before going to bed.

- Once you finish eating your food, it's advisable to lie down so the food and fluids in your stomach can be digested properly. Proper digestion reduces the risk of developing dyspepsia, so the chances of the acidic content flowing back into the esophagus are low.

- Tight-fitting attire may constrict the stomach and thus increase the chances of experiencing acid reflux. Avoid such clothes if you have GERD.

Over-the-Counter and Prescription Medications

GERD patients can choose from a wide range of medications to treat or manage the disorder. However, it's crucial to consult a doctor before you take any medication including over-the-counter medications. Here is a list of some useful medications for GERD patients.

- **Medications to neutralize stomach acid** – One of the best ways to alleviate the burning sensation caused by the acidic content of the stomach is to neutralize the acid. You can simply purchase antacids like Mylanta, Tums, and Rolaids from the local drugstore and use them for quick relief. However, you should keep in mind that you need other medications to heal inflamed or damaged areas of the esophagus.

- **Medications to reduce acid production** – Gastric acid is responsible for the burning pain experienced by GERD patients. The pain can be reduced by taking medications that reduce acid production. These medications are commonly known as **H-2-receptor blockers**. There are over-the-counter and prescription-strength H-2-receptor blockers. The most common ones include ranitidine, nizatidine, famotidine, and cimetidine. These medications may not act as fast as antacids, but they provide long-lasting relief. They can reduce the amount of acid produced in the stomach for a day.

- **Medications to block acid production and heal damaged esophageal tissues** – Damaged esophageal tissues cause discomfort which can be reduced using certain medications. Medications that can block acid production and heal damaged esophageal tissues are known as **proton pump inhibitors**. They are more powerful than H-2-receptor blockers. The most popular over-the-counter proton pump inhibitors include omeprazole (Zegerid OTC or Prilosec OTC) and lansoprazole (Prevacid 24 H). Prescription-strength proton pump inhibitors include lansoprazole (Prevacid), esomeprazole (Nexium), pantoprazole (Protonix), omeprazole (Prilosec, Zegerid), dexlansoprazole (Dexilant), and rabeprazole (Aciphex).

- **Medications to heal ulcers and relieve abdominal pain** – If you are experiencing pain in the abdomen, you can take ranitidine and other histamine receptor blockers to reduce the pain. Those suffering from GERD may develop ulcers due to increased levels of stomach acid. Proton inhibitors like omeprazole and pantoprazole can reduce abdominal pain and lower the risk of developing ulcers.

- **Medications to quicken gastric emptying** – If you have GERD and realize that the stomach emptying process is slower than usual, you can take domperidone and other gastric motility agents to quicken the process. Faster stomach emptying reduces the chances of experiencing acid reflux and promotes digestion.

- **Medications for strengthening the lower esophageal sphincter** – Certain medications like Baclofen may alleviate the symptoms of GERD by reducing the frequency of relaxations of the patient's lower esophageal sphincter.

The above medications may help GERD patients in different ways, but patients should be aware of the possible side effects when taking any form of medication. Excessive use of some antacids may cause various side effects including diarrhea and kidney problems. Those taking H-2-receptor blockers should know that some of these mediations may increase the risk of bone fractures and vitamin B-12 deficiency if used for a long time. Proton pump inhibitors might cause headache, diarrhea, vomiting, and vitamin B-12 deficiency. Also, excessive use of these medications can increase the risk of having hip fractures. Medications used to strengthen the lower esophageal sphincter may cause nausea and fatigue.

Natural Remedies

Aside from using dietary changes, lifestyle changes, and medications, GERD patients can also manage the disorder using various natural remedies. These remedies have the power to relieve the signs and symptoms of the disorder if utilized properly. Some of the recommended natural remedies are based on research, but others are not supported by any research to prove their effectiveness. Nevertheless, there are many testimonials from GERD patients who have tried these remedies and managed to relieve the signs and symptoms of the disorder. If you don't know the effects these remedies might have on your body and health condition, make sure you see a doctor for further advice on the matter. Your doctor could give you useful information regarding the effectiveness and safety of the natural remedies you may want to use to relieve the symptoms of GERD. Here are some widely-used natural remedies for GERD patients.

- **Lose some weight** – Being overweight or obese is linked to many health problems including acid reflux. The excess body weight increases abdominal pressure. When this happens, the pressure may force the acidic content of the stomach to leak or flow back into the esophagus. Research findings have revealed that GERD patients can alleviate the symptoms of this digestive system disorder and prevent its development by losing those extra pounds. If you think you need to lose some weight, try to engage in physical activities and avoid foods that increase your body weight.

- **Eat raw almonds** – One of the most effective ways of reducing the burning sensation caused by gastric acid is to neutralize the acid. Instead of using antacids that might cause side effects, eat some raw almonds if you can find them. Almonds are naturally alkaline, so they can easily neutralize stomach acid without causing undesired effects.

- **Drink aloe vera juice** – GERD patients can balance gastric content pH by taking alkaline agents like aloe vera. Just like raw almonds, aloe vera reduces the amount of acid in the stomach to prevent esophageal tissue damage. According to a 2015 study, decolorized and purified aloe vera juice may reduce acid reflux symptoms without causing any side effects.

- **Mix water (½ cup) with baking soda (1 teaspoon) and drink** – You may not like the taste of this solution, but it's worth trying if you are experiencing acid reflux. The mixture is an alkaline agent that can neutralize gastric acid. This solution has proven to be effective for many years, so there's no reason to doubt its effectiveness. Once the acid is neutralized, you will no longer experience the irritating chest pain and discomfort.

- **Eat an apple** – Generally, any food that acts as a neutralizing agent can reduce the effects of gastric acid when food flows back into the esophagus. Apples have alkaline properties that can neutralize gastric acid, so it's advisable to eat one after having your meal. Apples have a nice taste compared to aloe vera and baking soda, so you can have a bite, enjoy the taste, and benefit from the vitamins and alkaline properties.

- **Drink chamomile tea** – Research on chamomile and acid reflux has revealed that chamomile has antibacterial and anti-inflammatory properties. Acid reflux causes gastric acid to flow backward into the esophagus leading to painful inflammation in the esophagus. According to research findings, those experiencing this problem can benefit from the anti-inflammatory effects of chamomile. In theory, chamomile tea may reduce stress. Stress is a potential risk factor for acid reflux, so chamomile tea may reduce the effects of acid reflux.

- **Chew gum after meals** – Chewing gum may have several benefits for patients with GERD. The key benefit of chewing gum is that it makes your saliva more alkaline. Additionally, the salivary glands may produce more saliva when you are chewing gum. This means that you can swallow more saliva than usual. We already know that alkaline agents can neutralize the acidic content of the stomach. Therefore, chewing gum may soothe the esophagus and reduce inflammation.

- **Sleep on your left side** – One of the things you want to do if you are suffering from GERD is to prevent the acidic content of the stomach from moving backward into the esophagus during sleep. If you don't know what to do when the time to sleep comes, try to sleep on your left side. This will prevent the stomach acid from flowing back into your esophagus as you sleep. It also promotes the stomach emptying process during sleep even when lying down. In contrast, sleeping on the right side of your body can worsen the problem if you have GERD. It can also lead to delayed stomach emptying and you don't want this to happen if you are suffering from GERD.

- **Walk after a meal** – It's a well-known fact that physical activity is good for your health and overall wellbeing. When it comes to GERD management, you can promote digestion by having a short walk after meals. This is especially helpful after huge meals because it reduces the chances of having acid reflux. It prevents gastric acid from flowing back into your esophagus reducing the risk of having a damaged esophageal lining.

As you can see, GERD patients can easily manage the disorder by choosing from various treatments and management options. If you have GERD, there is no need to worry about it because you can manage it using your preferred option. Before you start the management or treatment process, it's important to monitor the signs and symptoms to know their characteristics and frequency. This is vital because it will help you take the appropriate action to lower the risk of developing complications. An accurate and timely diagnosis of GERD will also help you resolve the burning pain and discomfort as early as possible.

Of course, GERD patients are free to use over-the-counter medications, but it's always advisable to consult with your physician before you take any medication. You need to be sure that the drugs you intend to use will solve your problem without causing serious side effects. Whether you are taking over-the-counter or prescription medications, you need a doctor's advice. For patients who are already taking other drugs, it's necessary to know the possible side effects as well as adverse reactions before taking GERD medications. Some of the drugs might promote acid reflux and others may be the main cause of the problem. You may also be required to combine your GERD medications with other treatment options to achieve the best results.

The key to effective GERD management is to make dietary and lifestyle changes as well as take the recommended medications. You need to modify some of your lifestyle habits and avoid foods that might be responsible for your problem. When it comes to food and drinks, you should be aware of what is safe or not safe for consumption. Certain foods or drinks may contribute to high levels of acid in the stomach, but some healthy foods and drinks can neutralize the acid. If you drink alcohol or smoke cigarettes, limit your consumption because they will not only lead to GERD but also affect your overall health. Above all, you need to follow each of the recommended prevention steps if you want to lower the chances of developing GERD. If you address the risk factors in advance, then you don't have to look for treatment or worry about hospitalization.

Overall, there are reliable solutions for those suffering from GERD. You can manage the disorder at home as long as you know what to do. However, you should not wait for the condition to worsen without consulting a physician. You also need to see a doctor if you notice other unusual signs. If the doctor gives you instructions to manage GERD at home, make sure you follow each step faithfully. In any case, you want to avoid serious complications that might lead to hospitalization and expensive treatments.

Conclusion

Gastrointestinal tract health problems can be unpleasant because of the signs and symptoms associated with them. Patients with GI tract problems may vomit, lose appetite, feel nauseated, and experience intense abdominal pain. GERD is a common GI tract problem that can make life difficult for the patient. It's a digestive system disorder that affects 15 million individuals out of 60 million individuals every day. Fortunately, GERD is easy to manage and treat. There are many treatment options as well as natural remedies for relieving the signs and symptoms of GERD. With the right foods, drinks, lifestyle changes, and medication, those suffering from GERD can prevent the devastating effects of gastric acid. Generally, you can simply manage GERD by just making lifestyle and dietary changes.

Prolonged or untreated GERD can lead to various complications including esophageal strictures, tumors, ulcers, and cancer. Patients can prevent these complications from developing by starting treatment right away after an accurate diagnosis. Most GERD patients complain of heartburn, but other signs and symptoms need to be identified using laboratory tests and diagnostic procedures. An assessment is necessary to rule out other health problems.

It's not easy to live with GERD, but you can cope with the disorder by taking the appropriate steps. Make sure you track your acid refluxes and record their frequency and severity. If you have heartburns, keep records of their patterns so you can easily manage them even without seeing a doctor. If you don't know how to manage GERD at home, consult your physician and share your recordings of reflux episodes for further assistance. Modify your lifestyle habits and avoid potentially harmful foods and drinks as advised by your doctor. Switch to a balanced diet if you've been having unbalanced meals and take short walks after meals. Finally, remember to be patient and disciplined because it takes time and commitment to manage the signs and symptoms of GERD.

Paolo Jose de Luna

Printed in Dunstable, United Kingdom